Life After the Diagnosis

Life After the Diagnosis

Cindy Wiley

To order additional copies of this book, contact:
Xlibris Corporation
1-888-795-4274
www.Xlibris.com
Orders@Xlibris.com
96411

Contents

Foreward

Life After The Diagnosis is a journey of faith.

As you read through my story you will read times of despair, disappointment and discouragement. But I never lost my faith in God.

It was Him that brought be through those dark days and a great support system. You can't take this journey by yourself.

There is Life After The Diagnosis if you're willing to reach for it.

I have been blessed with a very creative mind that is always challenging me with the gifts and talents that God has given me. However, little did I know that when I was preparing to put "Cancer" baskets together for other caregivers and those that were going through chemo that I was preparing one for myself.

The journey through the diagnosis, surgery, radiation and chemo was awful, but I made it.

If I can offer these words of encouragement to anyone that has been diagnosed with cancer or is a survivor of this or any other debilitating disease that leaves you disabled even for a minute . . . never lose your faith in God.

It was God's grace, mercy and saving power that got me through such a horrible time. Prayers were going up for me from one side of the country to another including England—wherever I had friends but if I had lost my faith, I would have lost my life.

You know the scripture, "Faith is the substance of things hoped for, the evidence of things not seen. Hebrews 11:1 . . . that was me.

I prayed, I cried, I didn't understand why me, why now, but the Lord showed me all those answers in time. A lot of those whys were about me. There were areas of my life that needed corrected and I thank God that he gave me a second change. An opportunity to tell family I was sorry, rekindle an old friendship that I had not forgiven. Everything changed.

I do thank everyone for their prayers, visits, cards and other acts of kindness during that season. Words will never be able to express how I felt each time a phone call came although I couldn't talk, a card when I was so drugged I couldn't see straight, so weak that I couldn't lift my head, a touch of someone's hand. But TO GOD BE THE GLORY. I'm here and a survivor.

Don't take not one second of breath for granted. Thank God for every opportunity you get to open your eyes, to speak, to hear, to eat, to sing, to embrace your loved ones.

This book is dedicated to all cancer survivors and those going through. If you don't make it to through then you've made it to (resting until Jesus returns) and that's still ALL RIGHT!!

Acknowledgements

To my family, my daughter, grandchildren, nieces and nephews, sister-in-law and her extended family . . . thank you.

To Colette and Marsha who thought they were the "boss of me". Words will never express how I feel about the two of you. Always there for me, visiting, calling, holding my hand . . . Thank you

Crystal, Elder Wood, and Cheryl, thank you.

Rev. Lisa Winston, my mentor and my very special friend . . . thank you.

To my church family (Bishop Roberta Thomas, Pastor, and Fountain Gate Church & Ministries) thank you.

To Vickie Johnston, my sister in Christ, my friend. I will never be able to repay what you and Tae have done for me.

Compassionate Care Hospice where I learned so much about myself and what ministry was truly about.

Special Dedication
To My Sister Ruthie

What would have happened to me if my sister were not able to take me in? A nursing home, a hospice facility because my doctor thought I wouldn't make it? What?

Well, To God Be The Glory, it wasn't the case for me. Her name is Ruth (Dutch by our family nick name)

Just a little history about our relationship. Our mother passed away when I was two years old and she had to quit school to take care of me and my brother. From that time until this present day the bond between us has always been beyond any words that I could ever write or say. My confidante, my sister, my friend. Always there when I needed her.

I called her and asked her if I could come to live with her for a while because I had gotten so weak that I couldn't take care of myself. She agreed and I moved in with her, her daughter and grandson. What a time we had. They laughed at me when all I could do was drool and spit saliva using up toilet tissue and paper towels by the dozen. I killed a lot of trees. But it was always in love.

My great nephew, Jamar, came down one night and sat across from me and said "Aunt Cynthia" God is not finished with you yet". He read Psalms 40 to me. I shed some tears. First because he was only 15 at the time but so full of wisdom and I was so proud of him. Then for me because I was afraid but this scripture gave me peace.

How would I have made it without her singing, praying, laughing, and sometimes crying (where I couldn't see her) walking with me every step of the way to recovery. Always encouraging me when it was draining her to see her youngest sister in such a bad state. Through baby food, popcorn, root beer soda, cheese crackers, baked potatoes and so many other crazy foods. My taste buds were all over the place. But she always obliged me and told me she had to stay on her course because she was gaining weight with all the stuff I was eating. Channel 33, 42, 54, 64, 39. Our favorite channels every night for 7 months. We laughed every time we turned the channel. The little things.

She has two daughters and a son who passed away at an early age. She is a grandmother and great grand mother.

We share stories of our loved ones that have gone on. Stories of our parents and how they survived the depression, two floods with all 9 of us that survived out of 12. Yeah, my Dad believed in large families. We laugh and talk to this very day until the tears roll down our faces. What joy she brings into my life. There are only three of us left now but the memories we have. Make sure you're making memories for you and your loved ones. You only get one time.

She is a joy and sometimes has made me angry pushing me but only in love that she cared for me as only a sister that loves from her heart could.

It wasn't suppose to happen this way by man's perspective, because she's older and I'm younger. But God had a plan and we had to walk it out together. We did . . . we made it.

I dedicate much of my recovery time to her walking with me until I was 'cancer free' and back on my own again.

With all the love that I have within me, my sister . . . this is for you.

Love you

Tack

The Happening

It wasn't a normal day this day because I wasn't feeling well before I left for church . . . but I pressed. I had vomited some black stuff which I knew was old blood and had diarrhea which was also black. I knew I was bleeding somewhere but I wanted to get to church.

I got there but couldn't get any further than the back pew where I fell to the floor and couldn't move because I was so weak. I called to a member of the church that was passing by and informed her what was happening and asked her to keep me in prayer but I would just stay there because I couldn't move.

I made it through service (barely) and asked my cohort in crime to go with me to the emergency room. She agreed as always (we had previously done this January 09, and July 09 and November, 09)

When we got there you have to undress and put the ugly hospital gown on, get an IV, take 99 tubes of blood (just kidding), chest x-ray and stay put. Well, for me being a nurse is not always a good thing. I know some stuff plus I'm going to ask questions. It's just in me.

After thumping, probing and prodding, the Dr. came in and said Ms. Wiley, we need to give you 2 units of blood as your red count is down to 6 (normal is 12). I said ok because of my symptoms I knew I was bleeding somewhere. And also you'll be staying. Now he got my attention. Hate hospitals. People get sick there.

My cohort in crime (Vickie) called all of the appropriate people. She has a list with phone numbers, etc., and let them know what was happening and I would be going to a room and I think she liked seeing me not being in control.

My niece showed up (Colette) gave more information to the doctor. It wasn't nice of her to tell so much and we all said good night.

All throughout the night was more blood taking, more poking and prodding, and I never got any sleep. The next day they brought in 32 ounces of this orange stuff (taste like crystal light) right . . . and said you need to drink this because they are going to do a test tomorrow 1/26 to see what's going on down there. In other words, I had to be cleaned out. You got the picture. So, clear liquids, the orange stuff all day to the BR 20 times until clear. It didn't take much because I didn't have any food to eat. But who cared anyway the food was Yuk! The test is called a endoscopy . . . GOOD NIGHT

D Day

After not sleeping much during the night, by mid-morning 1/26, it was time for my test. They put you in a twilight sleep for the test and wake you up gradually when it's over.

By late afternoon they had their diagnosis D-Day. The entire team of doctors came into the room with solemn looks on their faces and my doctor spoke and said we have some bad news—you have gastric cancer.

I responded and said you've got to be kidding . . . I have things to do. We were supposed to be leaving for North Carolina for a conference (my cohort and myself). He said no . . . I'm sorry. What was he sorry about? I was the one receiving the Diagnosis. So I politely asked him to leave the room because I needed to cry and call my sister.

The day was filled with many phone calls to family. My daughter became angry. I don't think she knew how to handle her emotions.

My doctor came back and recommended surgery to remove the tumors and ask what surgeon would I like. I informed him which one. The surgeon came in and scheduled surgery for 2/2. He said 'I will get every bit of cancer I can'. Oh, I forgot they found an area on my Liver but it was negative (praise God)

More calls to family to keep them updated and the Pastor for prayer.

I just wanted to scream because of the unknown. Even with my medical background, I was not prepared for this for me. Was going to Compassionate

Care Hospice to work preparation for this? I cried more, read my word, asked for a sleeping pill to sleep but not for long.

They loaded me up with nutrients over the next several days, protein, and all kinds of stuff to get me built up. My stomach was going to be reduced to almost nothing after surgery and I would only be able to eat small meals several times a day. (What a way to lose weight)

My doctor informed me that I would be in ICU for about 2-3 days and then transferred back to a room.

The night before surgery, Pastor Crystal Lyde came to visit and we prayed so intensely that the security guard came in to make sure everything was all right. We cried and laughed at the same time as we knew that surgery is sometimes scary. My spirit was at peace.

After Surgery & ICU

Well, I made it through surgery after 5 hours and by my side was my niece, Marsha . . . waiting for me to wake up and give her a sign that I was o.k. Well, the doctor was right. I ended up in ICU for a few days on a respirator for a day (YUK)

If I ever needed my family, it was then because I was so scared. She stayed as long as she could (11:30 p.m.) but just the touch of her hand and although I couldn't see her face real clear, I knew she was there. Being the boss of me as usual. Telling the nurse I needed something for pain and caring and loving me as she does. What a blessing.

There were others that came. Some I remember, like my niece and her son. We had such a good time together that the ICU nurse said I needed to get out of there because we were having too much fun. Laughing to keep from crying. Oh by the way, the laugh I had would make anybody laugh. It wasn't a laugh but a sound that imitated a laugh. It had everyone cracking up.

A good friend Elder Wood, my friend Cheryl and others . . . I just don't remember because I was so drugged up.

The nursing staff was great . . . especially on night shift.

The tube finally came out only for me to find out that I had a nasal gastric tube in which I wanted to yank out but it all turned out well. After three days, they sent me to another room to begin my healing process in preparation to go home.

The NG tube came out about 2 days later and I was a happy camper. I didn't like the fact that I had to be put on a bed pan . . . sometimes I made it and sometimes I didn't (totally embarrassed) but it's part of the process.

PT/OT every day was a pain in the butt. However, if you want to go home, its what you have to do.

Another week in the hospital and it was time to go home. Thank God I didn't go home during all of that snow that took place at the beginning of February.

I stayed with my niece (Colette) for about a month . . . got pampered, good meals, good conversation and laughter about our family. Her Dad was my brother Bob who passed away several years ago.

The Pickle

One night because of my crazy appetite, I craved different things like when you're pregnant. My niece came up to use the computer and she was eating a dill pickle. I asked her for a piece and she told me "no". I thought I would have a fit because I could taste it in my mouth and it smelled really good. But she told me 'no'. We laughed but I still didn't get a piece. She had her daughter make me a grilled cheese sandwich the next day with a dill pickle on my tray. Love you Colette.

Radiation

After my return home, my first visit was to my surgeon and then my radiation oncologist. 25 rounds of radiation. YUK. I thought I would die. My color changed and my appetite left. It made me extremely weak. I met with a dietitian to increase my nutrients but nothing was working. I did the best I could.

One week I had radiation and chemo together . . . now that was awful. I was losing weight by leaps and bounds. I couldn't keep any food down, clothes were falling off me but I didn't want to eat or drink and just became weaker by the weeks. All I could do was sleep.

I hated going for these treatments watching others come in looking weak and weary as I did. What would there outcome be? I prayed for them as we always greeted each other every week as you got to know people.

It was hard on my best friend Vickie as she saw me losing the spark in my eyes, my steps slowing down and getting weaker by the days. She never said much at that time but since that time whenever we talk about it, we cry because I've come so far and we both remember when. I never want to be in that place ever again. TO GOD BE THE GLORY !!

I finished all my radiation treatments and now it was time for the dreaded "C"—CHEMO!

CHEMO—
How it changed
my life forever

There were all kinds of articles on Chemo but you can never read enough to get you through what you were going to experience. No one could help you. Medicine didn't help with the nausea and vomiting or with the diarrhea.

I tried several different medications and the only medication that worked for me was Ativan, Zofran and Phenergan suppositories. (yuk)

The Chemo weakened my immune system, I ran fevers constantly but at that time not enough to put me in the Hospital.

I was receiving Chemo 5 days a week, once a month. I had blisters inside my mouth, hair fell out, sleepless nights, night sweats, and aching bones, could barely walk, became dehydrated several times and had to have water via IV. Finally my white count dropped so low, my doctor had to admit me to the hospital. It was horrible. I had received two units of blood and shots to increase my white count. It all worked out. At that point my doctor indicated that the next 24-48 hours would be critical. I made it through.

I had finished my third round of chemo of 5 days. My doctor suggested that we do one more round of 5 days. I knew within myself that if God didn't give me the answer, I would die. I prayed all night long and when we went to the doctor's appointment, he said I'm not going to give you anymore Chemo and I would have said no any way because I was so weak my body couldn't take anymore.

That inner voice was still speaking to me telling me to get another opinion and I did. I switched oncologist and I haven't looked back since. I'm glad it wasn't too late. When you hear that inner voice, (which was the Holy Spirit) act on it.

I have a wonderful oncologist now and I'm so glad I switched. He's honest with me about my condition and explains everything, answers my questions and we are moving forward.

Don't be afraid to question medications, care plans or anything that affects your life. IT'S YOUR LIFE!!

I felt I was at death's door several times, but God pulled me through by His grace and His mercy!

I waited patiently for the Lord; and He inclined to me. And heard my cry. He also brought me up out of a horrible pit. Out of the miry clay. And set my feet upon a rock. And established my steps. Psalm 40:1-2

A Nursing Home Experience

I did have to do a month of rehab at one of the nursing home facilities in the area to get my stamina, walking, and eating back on track. I had Physical and Occupational Therapy every day. I wasn't the best patient. They say that about nurses and doctors. I hated it but it was worth it. That experience is one I won't forget for a long time.

I met some very nice people but the doctor that was in charge was one I could have done without. He wouldn't listen when I told him that the medication was making me hallucinate. I refused to take it and he became very belligerent with me. I stood my ground because you do have patient rights when you are in a facility.

He didn't like being questioned and certainly not challenged by a nurse telling him what you weren't going to do. Oh by the way, I also asked to see my chart. You have to be your own Advocate.

You won't believe it but he had made an entry that I needed a psych evaluation. If anyone needed a psych evaluation, it was him.

My nieces were by my side visiting just about every day. My daughter was still having difficulty seeing me in that condition and it was extremely hard for my grandchildren.

When I saw them cry one day, I knew I had to push harder to get better. I did everything PT/OT wanted me to do although I hated it. The therapy enabled me to go home.

God is my refuge and my strength; an ever present help in the time of trouble . . . Psalm 46:1

A New Beginning

If I could sum up everything that happened to me in 2010, it would go something like this. IT WAS HELL!!

Every fiber of my being was tested . . . doubt tried to overtake me about my God . . . I had to battle with depression, frustration, disappointment and anger on a daily basis, but my FAITH IN GOD kept me strong.

It was a journey that I hope whoever buys this book or gives it to someone else as a gift realizes that until you've walked in someone shoes that has gone through all of this, could only guess what it felt like. Just be there. Listen a lot as we tell our story over and over again. It helps with the healing process.

From walking out of my pants when I got too thin, sneaking to drive the car when I was supposed to be resting, eating in the middle of the night because I was hungry (peaches, sloppy joes, kielbasa and my favorite sauerkraut) yeah baby . . . it was a journey.

After I finished a month of rehab. I was on my way back. My sister made me walk every other day to the corner if I could or just sit outside to get fresh air. Friends from my job supplied me with a recliner so I could sleep by my self (it reclined to a very comfortable position) and I slept well. More incision pain as opposed to whatever pain I was supposed to have from the cancer. I never had any. (Hallelujah)

There is life after the diagnosis if you want it to be. I always pressed to go to church because I knew that was where my strength came from.

I know it was hard for the saints, family and friends to see me in the condition I was in but if they only knew how hard it was for me to see me that way as well.

Our God is a great God. When he says in his word "I'll never leave you nor forsake you", He meant it.

Be encouraging, laugh, cry, tell jokes, touch us . . . we're not contagious. We just have cancer.

I was ready to return to work in January, 2011 but not as a Hospice Nurse. I started sending out resumes. Of course it didn't help to be 62 looking for a job again but I just couldn't sit home collecting disability or work part time somewhere when I had a chance to live again.

I finally got an interview after several months of trying. I applied for a position as a Wellness Nurse but ended up getting the position of Program Director for the Memory Care Department. (Dementia/Alzheimer's) Only God!! I also no longer have Type 2 Diabetes.

Medical insurance coverage was another nightmare, COBRA was too expensive, and I couldn't get any help from Welfare. You had to be "Cancer Free" for 3-5 years to get any medical coverage from a broker. Welfare stated that I received too much money from Social Security. Can you imagine that? So from October until March I had no medical insurance coverage and prayed everyday that I wouldn't get sick. I made it.

Life after the diagnosis is a battle back and a journey but I made it and I'm so glad to still be alive. Never give up and fight every step of the way.

I'm on my own again and I'm only looking and moving forward. I'm blessed to be a blessing!! To God Be The Glory!!

Welcome to the poetry segment of the book that I have dedicated to women around the world. Be blessed!

The Woman Within ©

Words of
Encouragement & Inspiration

Cindy has been writing poetry since she was 10 years old.

She acknowledges Christ as the head of her life and the inspiration of her Mother and Father for her success.

The spirit of God has touched and blessed her life in so many ways. Her words capture the essence of someone's pain. She writes to encourage and inspire under the unction of the Holy Spirit. She's said on several occasions 'that if she tries to force words, it just doesn't work. All words are inspired from the Lord'.

She tells the story of her mother, now deceased, would listen to the radio and send a note of encouragement to people that were sick and needed encouragement if addresses were supplied. So I guess you could say that it was her purpose and destiny to become a writer and a poet from the time she was in her mother's womb.

To all of her sisters in Christ but most of all her biological sisters and her mother who made the supreme sacrifice—She honors you all and loves you.

She acknowledges the cost of the oil in their lives and what they have given to others.

She has been 'blessed to be a blessing' to others through the words God has given her. Her prayer is that these words will enhance your life, press you to that place in God and bring out "The Woman Within".

Cindy is the Founder of 'Sisters Overcoming Obstacles'©—Women Support Ministry, Seasoned Hearts©—Long Term Care Consultants/ Advocates, Babysitters Plus—Babysitting for Special Occasions, Extended Hands, Postpartum Doula Services and Inspirational Expressions by Cindy. All under the umbrella of "Touching Lives, Inc. Her ministries help her to minister to not only women but the family as a whole.

She was a Hospice Nurse, which made it so ironic when she got Cancer. She has been recognized for several of her poems by the International Society of Poets and has self published two books of poetry "Reflections"© and "The Journey"©. She also has a CD entitled "The Woman Within"©

She has a daughter Dawn, three grandchildren, Deija, Des'ree and Devon and a great granddaughter Ni Ni.

She has been a friend and an inspiration in my life.

—*Rev. Lisa Winston*

Poetry
Selections

The poem "The Woman Within"© was written for me during a very difficult time in my life by a dear friend and mentor Rev. Lisa Winston. With her permission I explored what I could do with the poem in written form and also on my CD entitled "The Woman Within"©.

It took me to a place where I could hear and see women from all walks of life that had and 'possibly' would experience all kinds of "stuff". I prayed and asked the Lord for some words to encourage their hearts for the pain, disappointment, betrayal, low self-esteem and just being "lost". He gave me the words within this segment. What I didn't realize at the time is I was writing that poetry for me. Not knowing that I would experience Cancer in the years to come (2010)

Do you recognize "The Woman Within"? Who she was, who she has become? The many paths she's traveled. Do you recognize her strength, her growth, her determination, and her brokenness? Do you see her joy, her peace, her defeats, and her success? Do you recognize her pain yet her deliverance? Could she be *you*? Could she be someone you know? Do you see her vulnerability, her dedication and commitment to God and family? Do you see *you*? Is there any greater gift than knowing who '**you**' are—and knowing whose you are in Christ?

Search and find "The Woman Within" for she is a mother, grandmother, sister, friend, cousin, aunt, niece, minister, co-worker, drug addict, an abused/abandoned woman, a prostitute, homeless, she has AIDS,—she is just a 'WOMAN'

The poems are dedicated to women around the world seeking to find 'The Woman Within'©.

This segment is dedicated to all the women who have blessed my life.—my mom, Edith Iona Miller (deceased), my daughter Dawn, my sisters—Iona (deceased), Regina (deceased), Ruthie, Rachel and all my sisters in Christ—I love you all!!

All That I Am

All that I am

I am because of thee

All that I'm not

Is because of me

—Anonymous

If It Is To Be

If it is to be, it is up to me

It is my choice, to think positively

Not negative or degrading things

How you think, is how you will be!

—Anonymous

Saving Me

Thank you Lord for saving me

And setting me on my path

For it had not been for you

I don't know where I'd be.

For all my sins, you cleansed me

For all my faults, forgave me

For all my trials, walked with me

But you never, ever left me.

Exodus 14:13 "Stand still and see
the salvation of the Lord . . . ."

Love Yourself

If you don't really love yourself

How do you think others will?

If you don't like the way you look

How do you think others feel?

When you look in the mirror

And can't see the beauty within

You can't blame anyone but yourself

You are your own best friend.

Love yourself no matter what

And no matter what others say

The gifts you have are yours alone

Use them to their fullest every day.

Often We Forget

Thank you comes rather easy

For people who are so kind

But this thank you comes

From deep within

Cause you've been on my mind;

Often we forget

To thank the ones who care

So thank you once for loving me

And thank you for always being there.

Hidden Treasure

As she hides within her house

The sounds begin to roar

The footsteps are getting closer

As she knows what is in store.

She hides her child beneath her

As they rip her world apart

A hand reaches out to console her

To help mend her wounded heart.

She is shunned by those she loves

Alone in her solemn place

The tears seem to be never ending

As they flow down from her face.

But deep within her spirit

A fire starts to burn

For all that she has been through

At each and every turn.

Through the eyes of others

She may be called disgraced

But in the eyes of the Master

She will always have a place.

Now when you see her

Her head is held up high

She is putting her life back together

Instead of wanting to die.

Although it will take time

To take away the pain

She will continue her fight onward

And never give up again.

They will **never** stop her from being

All she is to be!!

Prayerfully dedicated to the women in all of the African countries.

If It Had Not Been For You

If it had not been for you

I don't know where I would be

If it had not been for you

I would not have true liberty.

If it had not been for you

I would never have a chance

To see the doors opened in my life

With each and every glance.

If it had not been for you

I might not be here today

But because of your love for me

You took time to show me the right way.

If it had not been for you

I would certainly be lost

But because of what you've put in me

There is always a cost.

If it had not been for you

My father, my comforter, my friend

Satan would have had his way

And my life would have come to an end.

You took a piece of clay

And shaped me into who I am

You blew your breath of life into me

And now I can truly stand.

Thank you for your mercy

Thank you for your grace

It's in you I always want to dwell

And always seek your face.

So if it had not been for you

There would certainly be no me

In all I do I give you praise

For my purpose and my destiny.

Shattered Tears

Have you ever wondered

What it takes to form a tear

It could be thoughts of sadness

Or wasted painful years.

Shattered tears are different

They're gathered from your soul

A loved one loss

A friendship gone

A life out of control.

Shattered tears are memories

That keep you bound within

Shattered tears are heartaches

That have haunted you time and again.

As these tears roll down your face

Gods' hands are open wide

To catch each shattered tear you've shed

To place them within Him deep inside.

Within His heart filled with His love

For you His special one

For shattered tears is what He felt

For His one and only son.

Shattered tears bring cleansing

A renewing of who you are

You must let go of the past

For you have come so far.

Into this new beginning

Of all that God wants you to be

For shattered tears is just a part of life

That has shaped your destiny.

Their Eyes

Their eyes tell a story

Of the pain they have within

Their words pierce your heart

When they say, "I don't need friends".

Their eyes say please help me

"I don't know what to do

I don't know who to turn to

To help me make it through."

Their eyes say I want a chance

To be the best I can be

Their eyes tell a story

That someone has been touching me.

Someone has betrayed their trust

And ripped their world apart

Someone has taken their delicate soul

And broken their tender heart.

They're too young to have such problems

Children are suppose to have fun

Their world should be filled with laughter

Not frightened, scared or on the run.

They wanted to share this poem

So we would understand

That children in this environment

Need a helping hand.

To rebound from their heartache

To be normal once again

To learn to love themselves

To trust and to make good friends.

Dedicated to those who have been scarred and wounded by rape, molestation and abuse.

I Have More In Store

I have more in store for you

To walk in who you should be

I have more in store for you

I've given you my word to be free.

I have more in store for you

Not church like it used to be

But more of a revelation of who I am

And how close you should be to me.

The oil of my precious anointing

The fragrance of my spirit upon thee

I have more in store for you

Just press to me and you'll see.

All of the beauty and splendor

Of spending time with me

All that I plan to give you

Is here in the holy of holies with me.

I have more in store for you

To cast out what is not like me

The power, the dominion,

The authority to declare

That this is true victory.

So walk my blessed beloved

In all that He wants you to be

For He knows the plans He has for you

And has shaped your destiny.

Jeremiah 29:11 "For I know the thoughts that
I think toward you, says the Lord,
thoughts of peace and not of evil,
to give you a future and a hope.

A Helping Hand

We all need a helping hand

To help us on our way

When times are rough and rocky

We need someone to say.

I may not understand your sadness

And I may not understand your pain

I extend a helping hand

To help whenever I can.

We might need some kind words

To comfort and lift our souls

As life with all its changes

Sometimes can take its toll.

So, if I see you frowning

Or hanging your head down low

I extend a helping hand

To walk with you wherever you go.

And no, it won't be easy

As I may need your hand sometime

But that's okay hands are free

Like friendship, yours and mine.

The Shadow People

Lord, I can't believe

The hunger everywhere

The shadow people know

As they wonder here and there.

They take all that they have

In search of food and rest

But all they find is barren land

They've tried to do their best.

Their bellies are so swollen

Their bodies racked with pain

You see it's been so long for them

They just can't take the strain.

A child dies in their arms

A sister then a brother

No food has taken away their lives

And yes, even a father and mother.

So when you stop to pray

Think of them in their barren land

I wish it wasn't this way for them

Sometimes it's hard to understand.

*Dedicated to the hungry, impoverished people
around the nation*

A Smile

A smile can make you happy

When things are going wrong

A smile can say how much you care

And help to keep you strong.

A smile can fill a room

With laughter, joy and tears

A smile can be a memory

Of cherished, precious years.

A smile can say how are you?

I missed our talk today

A smile can touch a broken heart

And help you on your way.

A smile can ease sadness

Deep within your soul

A smile can stop tears from falling

When life is out of control.

The next time you feel unhappy

Just look in the mirror and see

What a pretty, precious smile you have

And it's all yours, wouldn't you agree?

I'm Grateful

Lord, I'm so grateful

For all you've done for me

I didn't know where I was headed

I didn't know where I might be.

My life was filled with confusion

Frustration and discontent

I wondered and worried for years

As I didn't know what faith really meant.

I even questioned the blessings

That followed me through the years

I couldn't understand

Why the Lord didn't answer my prayers.

Now when I look back

On the things I asked Him to do

I understand when there was silence

He was carrying me through.

I'm glad I found a Savior

Who's thoughtful and so kind

He never makes a mistake

And is always right on time.

Leading The Way

You don't need to know

Where you're going

If God is leading the way.

You don't need to know

Will I make it?

If you trust Him

And pray every day.

You don't need to know your future

For God will never let your fall

He promised never to forsake you

He promised to be there when you call.

Help Me To Heal

Help me to heal the sorrow

The pain I feel within

Help me to heal the heartache

That haunts me over and over again.

Help me to heal the hurt

As the tears roll down my face

Help me handle the disappointment

As I continue to run this race.

A healing touch is what I need

To help to get me through

I lay myself now at your feet

For true healing must come from you.

The Mask

When you look behind the mask

Who do you really see?

Is this the person you truly are?

Or someone everyone thinks you should be.

The mask can cover your sorrow

And also cover your pain

Yet once you remove the mask

You must face 'you' again.

The mask can cover many things

But will never cover who you are

Remove your mask and love yourself

For God made you a winner, a star.

Something Special About A Pastor

There's something special about a Pastor

They carry the care of their flock

There's something special about a Pastor

They wear a 24-hour clock.

There's something special about a Pastor

They also bear our pain

They also cry when loved ones die

And try to comfort the ones that remain.

The Lord placed in this person

The vision, the direction the course

He also gave them wisdom

To be still and to hear His voice.

When you leave on Sunday morning

And you shake your Pastor's hand

Take a minute to encourage them

And pray for them every chance that you can.

Sisters

Sisters are special people

Not just sisters but also friends

Sisters share many secrets

And are there for you time and again.

Sisters laugh and cry

And warm each other's hearts

Sisters make sacrifices

And always play their part.

Sisters are so special

A mother to a motherless child

Sisters can brighten a cloudy day

As you sit and chat for a while.

I wouldn't trade my sisters

For anything you see

Because all of my sisters are special

And helped me the best I can be.

Friends

Have you ever wondered

Where you'd be without your friends

The one you always call upon

Whose memory never ends.

They somehow always manage

To know when you're in need

The love you share is special

As you are friends in deed.

They become part of your family

Like a sister or a brother

And you wonder to yourself sometime

Why you don't get tired of each other.

Friends are quite a blessing

Like Jesus is to you and me

The next time you are together

Say thank-you for letting me be me.

The Woman Within

No one knows all the ins and outs

No one knows all your pains and doubts

No one knows the hurt behind the grin

No one but Jesus knows the woman within.

The woman outside is strong and sure

She knows what to do and when to do it

She has no doubts is assertive and sharp

But no one but Jesus knows the pain in her heart.

On her knees every night she spends time with her God

She laughs, she cries, she moans, she fights

She ask why me Lord, please help me to survive

Then the Lord comforts and strengthens the woman inside.

You're there for a reason I've chosen this place

This temple is in ruins, the people are disgraced

I need you to stand against evil and sin

I'm placing my power in the woman within

So go forth my dear daughter don't get tired or weak

I'm here when you need me my guidance too seek

Go forth my sweet solider, I'm there to the end

Just hold to the spirit of the woman within.

Thank you for purchasing 'Life After The Diagnosis"© which includes poems from "The Woman Within".

Please pray for women around the world that are not 'yet' free to learn to write, pray, and just be who they are in God but have been hindered because of slavery or bondage or 'inward turmoil. A diagnosis doesn't have to be health related, it can be life related that can push you to bad health.

'To God Be The Glory' for all that He has done and all that He is going to do.

When you decide to have a pity party for yourself consider this . . . . I had a mini-stroke in January 2009 and was informed that I had Type 2 Diabetes. July 2009 I had another mini stroke. I had my gallbladder out in November, 2009. If I ever needed to find 'The Woman Within' it was when I received the news about the cancer diagnosis. But I am still standing. I had no after effects after the two strokes and all I can say is 'Praise God.'

I thank God for the opportunity to share this with all of you so that you realize what a powerful, faithful, loving, caring and God answering prayer we serve. He loves you all so much. His will is the way to go for your life. You might not like it, but it will be worth it if you trust him. What He has done for me, He will do the same for you.

He has to get the glory out of your life.

Please continue to keep me in your prayers!!

Nothing is impossible for God!!

For speaking engagements, please contact me at (717) 343-2844 or via e-mail: *cindywiley@hotmail.com*

Cindy Miller-Wiley

www.ingramcontent.com/pod-product-compliance
Lightning Source LLC
Chambersburg PA
CBHW021911170526
45157CB00005B/2045